A.D.D.

The Natural Approach

Help for Children with Attention Deficit Disorder and Hyperactivity

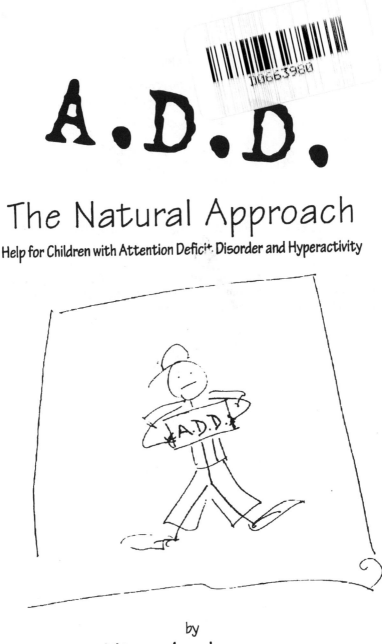

by
Nina Anderson
Howard Peiper

illustrated by
Rachel Bell

Twelfth Printing - July 1998
Printed in the United States of America

Published by Safe Goods
283 East Canaan Rd., East Canaan, CT 06024
(860)-824-5301

"A.D.D. The Natural Approach" is not intended as medical advice. It is
written solely for informational and educational purposes. Please consult a
health professional should the need for one be indicated.

SAFE GOODS
(860)-824-5301 FAX 824-0309

Table of Contents

A Note From the Author

For seventeen years now, my daughter has gathered information about natural healing methods. She started from scratch and learned through experimentation, formal apprenticeship, and by visiting and conversing with numerous professionals in alternative fields. She also worked in an instructive and supervisory capacity with adolescents clinically diagnosed with Attention Deficit Disorder and Hyperactivity.

Most of her students with ADD were taking medication. Those not receiving medication were unaware of alternative natural therapies for ADD, but were very interested in such things.

This booklet is for them, a token of appreciation to those blessed dreamers who reawakened her to the awesome potential and possibilities in life, and who, through their own outrageous imaginations, taught her to think big again.

Thank you Rachel for all you've done, and for all your support and encouragement, and thank you especially for holding the vision for this work and for seeing this first step through. We could not have done this without you!

Foreword

Attention Deficit Disorder - Welcome to the 21st Century

The number of children labeled hyperactive or learning disabled has reached epidemic proportions. These children with non-compliant behavior have no obvious cause of disease to be found by physical examination or laboratory tests. The quick cookbook response for the problem is usually a behavior modifying drug called Ritalin, as popular today as Tylenol or aspirin.

The answer for hyperactivity can be very simple, but is not an easy one. To me hyperactivity, as any other serious chronic problem, is a sign of toxicity or deficiency or, most of the time, a combination of both. The child with brain disorder is the same one who more than likely was not breast fed, was colicky or constipated when given formulas, and had gastro-esophagal reflux for which he or she was given Tagamet or Zantac. It is also the child who has been on multiple antibiotics for ear infection or throat infection. It is the same child who does not sleep well at night or who has frequent stomach aches or leg aches, is always congested and gets every single cold that comes around. And it is the child that is very frequently diagnosed as an asthmatic very early in life and is taking Albuterol and Prednisone.

If the nose is stressed out it runs, if the lungs are stressed out they wheeze or cough, if the stomach is stressed out it aches. When the brain is stressed out it will produce, not a rash, but a distorted thought, an inappropriate feeling, or an inaccurate perception. Ritalin helps a few children in the short run, but it is clear that it is not the answer for the long run. We, in the health field, have to find the real solution: modification of our internal and external environment, removing toxicity, cleaning our digestive system, improving immunity and liver detoxification. We have to properly feed our brain by improving our diet and by paying more attention to our intake of essential fatty acids and amino acids. Mineral intake is very much neglected nowadays. The time for a more natural and holistic approach to treating children with brain disorders is more than overdue.

5

Parents, teachers, health professionals and the children will appreciate your contribution. Welcome to the 21st century.

— *Esteban A. Genao, M.D., F.A.A.P.*
pediatrician

"ADD and ADHD are not diseases or disorders in the orthodox sense. The sufferers of these conditions are mal-adjusted, mal-nourished, impaired by abnormal brain chemistry, and most often our society is the cause. We feed our children nutritionless pseudo-foods, artificial colors, preservatives and allergens (wheat, dairy, etc.). We sit them in front of the constant changing and stimulating images of television and video games. Then we expect them to sit quietly throughout the school day. Everything is tightly scheduled; never enough time for sleep, unregulated play, real relaxation and time to be human.

In my opinion, ADD (and ADHD) are the result of people trying to live machine lives in machine-time; the end product of an inhuman(e) left-brain, linear cultural society leaving no room for round pegs in very narrow square holes. Our society's answer: Prozac, Cylert and Ritalin - the medicated life! The alternative to "better living through chemistry" is to slow down, sleep more, eat "real" foods, change the way we educate our children (the Steiner schools are a wonderful model), and enjoy life - a real life - not televised images of life-out-of-balance. Use herbs and nutrients to strengthen the nervous, circulatory and endocrine system. If this doesn't work (or you don't have the time) the prescription for Ritalin is always available."

— *David Winston, Herbalist, Ethnobotanist,*
Co-founder of The American Herbalists Guild

"A major contributing factor to A.D.D. is cellular toxicity, specifically chemicals and metals. These toxins interfere with cellular function and repair. Therefore, we need to detoxify the body at a cellular level, to clean and strengthen the foundation before rebuilding nutritionally. A.D.D. can be corrected."

— *Gregory S. Ellis, Ph.D.*
Certified Nutrition Specialist

The Problem

More than 6 million American children take Ritalin regularly to help them with Attention Deficit Disorder (ADD), an increase of two and a half times since 1990. This statistic is conservative by some estimates. It seems everyone knows someone whose child is on a prescription for ADD or who is being advised to consider it.

Parents seeking solutions to their child's distractible, disruptive, and inattentive behaviors may be encouraged to medicate their children before other options have been explored, and doctors and school personnel may lead parents to believe that medication is the best or, in some cases, perhaps the only answer. Also, teachers are gaining the power in some school districts, to demand medical intervention for children who are disruptive. These tactics can leave parents with little or no choice but to medicate. Even nursery school teachers are encouraging parents to consider Ritalin for their preschool aged children.

Doctors may encourage the use of Ritalin because the results of "successful" Ritalin therapy are dramatic. When Ritalin does what it is "supposed" to do, a child who could not previously sit still or pay attention, suddenly becomes able to do both, seemingly overnight. While this may be impressive, it should never be considered a long term solution. A long term solution will be one that restores balance rather than simply masking the symptoms of imbalance.

When Ritalin is unsuccessful, there is no peace. A child may become violent or excessively irritable and impossible to communicate with. Some children become withdrawn and depressed, unable to laugh or play. If the family has no information about alternatives, despair may be the result.

Alternatives to Ritalin *do* exist. If Ritalin or another drug like it has failed in your child's case or if you prefer to go "all natural" there are time tested ways of doing so that you are about to discover.

Attention Deficit Disorder (ADD), and Attention Deficit Hyperactive Disorder (ADHD), are closely linked. It is most common these days to refer to ADD *with* hyperactivity or ADD *without* hyperactivity.

In any case, the problem results from a disturbance of the central nervous system, and most experts now agree that ADD is a brain disorder with a biological basis.

In the past it was thought that children displaying the behaviors of ADD were brain damaged, hence the name "minimal brain dysfunction" was applied for a time. Then "hyperkinesis" became the label of the day, soon followed by "attention deficit disorder" and "attention deficit hyperactive disorder." There is always discussion as to what a more appropriate name for this "disorder" may be.

Sentiment leans towards replacing the "deficit disorder" in "attention deficit disorder" with something more appropriate. That is to say that often, rather than a deficit of attention, there is an abundance of attention (in too many directions), alternating with the ability to hyperfocus at times.

ADD sufferers normally have average or above average intelligence, and may be superbly gifted. Albert Einstein, Thomas Edison, and Henry Ford all did poorly in school; Einstein was expelled. Also, the "deficit" of attention seems to disappear when the intensity of interest in a thing takes over.

Supposedly there is no known cure for ADD, but remember — ADD is a manifestation of symptoms traceable to the central nervous system and to an imbalance thereof; if balance is restored to this system, then the symptoms of ADD should improve, and they do, and there are a variety of ways to accomplish this.

What About Ritalin?

Very little is known about how Ritalin works or why, and its long term safety is of yet undetermined.

Ritalin is a class II drug, defined as a controlled substance and categorized with cocaine, methadone, and methamphetamine.

Class II drugs are noted for their "high abuse potential"; however, proponents of the drug argue that Ritalin is harmless in therapeutic doses. They support their opinions by citing cases where children have experienced tremendous improvement in their symptoms while on the medication. While this may be true, one must also weigh the potential consequences.

Ritalin has many possible severe side effects. Because the connection between the side effects and the medication is often overlooked, years may be spent treating insomnia, or rash, or excessive irritability, and so forth when the real culprit is the prescription drug the child is taking. Girls, especially, are subject to being treated for the side effects of Ritalin or other drugs like it. Often their menstrual periods are blamed or their "inherent tendency", or their "extreme sensitivity".

Even where Ritalin appears to benefit the patient, dosages may need to be "upped" regularly as tolerance builds. And although tolerance and addiction often go hand in hand, proponents of Ritalin scoff when addiction is mentioned as a possible risk factor. Doctors who prescribe Ritalin say the therapeutic dosages are so extremely minute that the risk of hard core addiction is virtually impossible; this may or may not be true.

But the matter of addiction aside, it is still worth noting that a gradual period of withdrawal is recommended. One should never stop the medication suddenly. Severe depression and serious other side effects may result as a consequence of premature withdrawal from Ritalin or other drugs like it.

Never discontinue the medication without first consulting the physician who prescribed it.

A Doctor's Reference

It has been more than a decade since Dr. Robert Mendelsohn, M.D., author of *How to Raise a Healthy Child in Spite of Your Doctor* explicitly warned parents against the use of Ritalin and similar drugs, yet in that time Ritalin sales have skyrocketed. Why? Have we so lost sight of our natural roots and rhythms so as to be unable to recall the importance of sufficient rest, relaxation, and faith in the natural world as it pertains to our health? Compassion and wisdom, contemplation, meditation, innate knowledge, human love and understanding, nourishment from the earth — these are the real healers. Mendelsohn understood this many years ago.

Dr. Mendelsohn was a conventional pediatrician for over twenty years practicing orthodox medicine. He ordered x-rays, tonsillectomies and other routine therapies that he later came to regard as unnecessary. Gradually, Mendelsohn's beliefs shifted and he began encouraging people, especially parents, to rely more on their own 'judgment and ability to fare and to place less emphasis on "doctor's orders." His first two books: *Confessions of a Medical Heretic* and *Male Practice: How Doctors Manipulate Women,* caution readers about the hazards of blind faith in the medical professions. His third book: *How to Raise a Healthy Child in Spite of Your Doctor* encourages parents to take the power of caring for their children back into their own hands.

Mendelsohn says that parents and grandparents are more capable than doctors of managing the health of young children. He warns against the use of drugs for behavior modification and insists that parents must search for the underlying causes of erratic behavior. Regarding Ritalin and other drugs like it, Mendelsohn counsels parents to reject these drugs "out of hand," insisting there are no benefits to the children that are worth the risks.

Why Go Natural?

Learning disabilities can be caused by genetic defects or by metabolic disorders. In the case of genetic defects, the learning disability is connected to mental or physical defects that can lead to serious conditions, such as idiocy and cannot be changed by any known therapy. Many of these learn disabilities are not caused by genetic defects, but by metabolic disorders originating immediately after birth or even caused by the mother's physical condition during pregnancy. To understand what is happening in these cases, we have to understand how the body and the brain function.

All tissues in the body, including the brain and nerves, are composed of cells which are complete entities and interconnected with all other cells in the body. Each cell sustains its own metabolism and many perform tasks beneficial to the whole body. This process depends on over 2000 enzymes produced by the cells. If enzymes are destroyed by toxins which have been introduced into the body through the air, water and the food we eat, metabolic functions will be impaired, causing a malfunction in body processes. Many babies are born with toxins derived from the mother, and during the early stages of life more may accumulate due to ingesting food containing pesticides, chemicals and additives.

The brain and nerves are vulnerable, because toxins interfere with enzymatic function need to preserve proper metabolic operation. Deficiencies in this area can cause mood swings, attention span problems, hyperactivity and deterioration in health. Eventually the lack of enzymatic function will prevent proper digestion resulting in malabsorption of nutrients, further complicating the problem. Classical medical treatment does not address the problem correctly. In the case of learning disabilities, several factors interact. The child with a fragile genetic makeup is vulnerable to many types of toxins which may not be eliminated properly due to a malfunctioning or congested liver. Natural methods of cleansing the body and removing the toxins are a powerful way to treat this "illness."

Gregory Ellis, Ph.D., is a Certified Nutrition Specialist. He has developed a specific program for ADD that considers cellular toxicity as a predisposing or contributing factor in the disorder. His program begins with a clearing of all eliminative organs and follows with specific cellular detoxification for chemicals, metals and viruses. He employs homeovitic formulations to accomplish this cellular cleansing. Nutritional rebuilding is then initiated, much like rebuilding a house on a stronger, clean foundation. This process has worked successfully on autism as well.

> *"Go on, be free, and wake up singing."*
> — Olivia Franklin

Natural therapies support the body's innate ability to heal itself. Nature always finds balance, and balance is what we strive for in a natural way of life. Balance is what natural therapies seek to restore. And in a sense this is our constant and undeniable answer for all time — to find balance.

When we eat fresh, organic grains, fruits, and vegetables; when we breathe fresh air, drink pure water, and think pure thoughts we are giving our body a way to be healthy and free, and we are giving ourselves and our children the gift of a quality life.

Nourishment is offered through herbs and minerals. Laughter is good medicine. Guided imagery, massage, aroma therapy, acupuncture, chiropractic, hypnotherapy, yoga, and many other modalities all have the potential to relieve stress, and promote health and well being. Yet we must be patient and understand that sometimes healing takes a lot of time.

And although the "natural way" may at times be more difficult than you might have imagined, stick with it and discover this path's truly awesome rewards.

Nutrition, The Common Sense Therapy

In an astounding article entitled *Why are Kids Killing Kids* I. Gerald Olarsch, N.D. discusses the consequences of mineral deficiency as it relates to our children and American society. Dr. Olarsch links hyperactivity and learning problems, and violent behavior to a fundamental lack of minerals. Dr. Olarsch insists that attention deficit disorder and hyperactivity — among other abnormal behaviors — may be serious indicators of a lifetime of potentially worsening hardships, including depression and instability. If we look at so many cases of attention deficit disorder we see that these children often have had more health and behavior problems than others. Chronic ear infections, colic, and irritable behavior are common in these children. Usable, assimilable, healthful minerals are in critically short supply or nonexistent in American soils and aqueducts. Our sources of drinking water are questionable at best and polluted on the average. This, however is only part of the problem. The consumption of refined sugar, refined salt, chemical dyes, artificial flavorings, and empty calorie meals are detrimental to our health. It is not a matter of debate anymore, it is a fact.

Dr. Olarsch tells us about the behavior known as pica, a severe and obsessive craving for foods due to mineral deficiencies. It appears most commonly in children as an extreme desire for sugary and salty foods, This, Dr. Olarsch says, is because, "Unfortunately for us our body temporarily translates sugar and salt consumption as a fulfillment of the craving for nutritional minerals. Low iron levels were found to impair judgment, reasoning ability, and all aspects of left brain activity, including scientific, mathematical, and spoken and written language skills."

Another ramification of long-term mineral deficiency is that the body will latch on to heavy metals in an attempt to satisfy itself. If the body has no minerals available that are good for it, the body will instead latch on to and store excess lead, aluminum, copper and the like — whatever it is exposed to. On the other hand, when good minerals are available, the body will be able to choose the good over the bad.

One study positively linked high copper levels in the brain to violent behavior in boys in a detention home. Every subject in the study showed high copper levels. What the study did not discuss was how to correct the problem for although it is unhealthy to be overloaded with copper or other metal contaminants, it is not irreversible. Taking liquid crystalloid electrolyte minerals will alleviate this problem and help to chelate (get rid of) existing heavy metal deposits in the body.

This is not to say that children with ADD are prone to violence per sé. But what is the connection between malnutrition or mineral deficiency and aberrant behavior? Isn't it interesting that a majority of hardened criminals suffered from learning disabilities, hyperactive behavior, malnutrition and the like. Somewhere we have to begin to make a connection.

Trace Minerals

The Vilcabambas tribe and the Hunzas are people known for their long, vibrantly healthy lives. Both drink highly mineralized water.

What appears to be the chief reason for good health, and mineral balance is attributed to their mineral-rich waters, and especially its content of the very minerals that are most missing, or dangerously low, in most commercial and public waters.

The Vilcabambas as do the Hunzas, drink mineral rich water from mountain streams which flow underground and on the surface, over rocky formations which release not only calcium, but all other minerals and trace-elements as well. Electrically charged, positively or negatively, from the friction of flowing and tumbling waters unpolluted, they provide readily available, unpolluted, and assimilable minerals.

Minerals nourish our cells bringing forth vitality and a childlike sense of wonderment. Lack of minerals causes a grim outlook on life and leaves us prone to degenerative disease, and a host of mental and emotional ills. Minerals must be taken in an easily assimilable form such as a crystalloid formula. A crystalloid formula provides minerals that can pass through cell walls and do their work on a microscopic level enabling the whole system to function more effectively.

Absolutely everyone can benefit from taking liquid electrolyte crystalloid minerals, but for kids with attention deficit disorder it is not only indicated, it is essential.

Magnesium

Another possibly widespread deficiency involves magnesium. Clinically low levels of magnesium in blood plasma are associated with states of hyper-excitability and inattention in children. Mildred Seelig, executive director of the American College of Nutrition estimates that 80 to 90 percent of children are magnesium deficient.

Zinc

Zinc deficiency has been linked to certain behavioral problems including ADD. One Florida pediatrician, Estaban Genoa, M.D. has had tremendous success treating ADD in children with supplements of liquid electrolyte trace minerals and extra zinc. Oddly enough, zinc is a cofactor in numerous enzymatic processes and reactions, and enzymes, as we know, are essential not only to health, but to life itself. It seems to follow that a deficiency of zinc would automatically inhibit certain enzymatic functions — whatever they may be — and that this is perhaps a very key and basic element of the clinical picture of attention deficit disorder, and may in fact be one reason why taking enzyme supplements aids in the healing of the symptoms of ADD — because the extra enzymes make up for a chronic deficiency of zinc. This is only speculation, but probably worth considering. Perhaps by now you are beginning to see how these pieces of the puzzle — minerals, enzymes, EFA'S, — relate to one another, how they are all so intertwined as to really be inseparable parts of one whole system. One doctor told me that once zinc has become deficient, it takes three generations for the problem to correct itself. Dr. Genao gets fabulous results with children taking zinc supplements and liquid trace minerals for ADD along with making certain changes in the diet. Zinc dosages must be carefully prescribed according to the weight and condition of the person.

Enzymes

Enzymes digest food and aid in tissue repair, they are the construction workers of the body; life depends on them. The body manufactures a limited supply of enzymes for the purpose of digestion, and what other enzymes are required must be supplied from the foods that we eat. But there's a catch — only raw foods contain enzymes, cooked and processed foods do not. Therefore a child who consumes a diet mainly of cooked and processed foods is at a high risk for developing enzyme deficiency and its related symptoms. These may be anything from digestive upset to chronic irritability and fatigue to early signs of degenerative aging including *impaired mental capacity*. Studies have been done to prove that cooked foods alone cannot sustain life.

Without enzymes the biological process breaks down. This weakens the immune system and all other bodily functions. Enzyme deficiency has also been shown to promote food allergies due to improper digestion and this can contribute to behavior anomalies.

Obtaining enzymes for personal use is simple. The most desirable enzymes for supplementation are plant enzymes. These come in capsules and in powdered form to be used by the teaspoon and taken either directly into the mouth (the taste is sweet) or sprinkled onto food. Enzymes must be taken every time cooked or processed food is eaten. Begin supplementation in small doses. The benefits may include: improved digestion, feeling less sleepy after meals, enhanced clarity of thought (more energy going to the brain and less to digesting processed food), and improved overall functioning.

Essential Fatty Acids

Essential Fatty Acids (EFA's) are incredibly simple to obtain and can make a noticeable difference in one's health if taken on a regular basis. The most fortunate among us received EFA's from our mother's breast milk if we were nursed as infants. This helps the baby's brain develop the way it is supposed to. The curious thing about EFA's is that they must be obtained from outside food sources since the body cannot make them. Found in high concentrations in the brain, EFA's aid transmission of nerve impulses and are needed for normal brain functioning — this is their direct connection to treating children with ADD. EFA's — also referred to as Omega-3's or Omega-6's — are indicated for children and adolescents with ADD because **EFA's are food for the brain.**

Evidence states that the infants of mother's who were sufficiently supplied throughout their pregnancies with essential fatty acids are brighter and learn faster. Yet all is not lost if EFA's have been lacking in the diet even since birth. It is possible to supply these nutrients now and still enjoy the benefits, and in a relatively short period of time.

Flax meal and borage oil are the best sources for children. Borage oil may be taken in the capsule form. Flax meal is a food supplement that may be sprinkled on salads, soups, and cereal. Flax meal has a pleasant, nutty flavor.

Proanthocyanidins

In the February 1995 issue of *Total Health,* Willa Vae Bowles told the story of a little girl from Kalamazoo, Michigan who in the first grade displayed hyperactivity, out-of-control behavior and declining schoolwork. The girl was diagnosed with ADD and Ritalin was prescribed. Although her schoolwork improved, the girl suffered some side effects from the medication including a nervous twitch and a terrible attitude. The doctor felt it unwise to continue the medication, but could offer no alternatives. The girl's mother prayed for guidance. In November 1993 the girl began taking Pycnogenol, one source of proanthocyanidin, and within three days there was a complete turnabout. The girl became calm and pleasant and was able to function harmoniously.

The reason this supplement is so effective is because Proanthocyanidins are super powerful antioxidants with the ability to cross the blood brain barrier. This may occur instantaneously and be very noticeable. When this happens, heating takes place. The result is more balance and clearer thinking.

Proanthocyanidins are substances found in grape skins, grape seeds, cranberries, blueberries, blackberries, red wine, red cabbage, apple skins, strawberries, and black cherries. They are the precursors to red, blue, and violet color pigmentation in plants. Proanthocyanidins are also found in select pine bark. The most popular sources for concentrated Proanthocyanidin supplements are Grape Seed Extract and Pycnogenol, an extract of French maritime pine bark or grape seed extract. Grape Seed extract is less expensive, more popular in Europe, and very effective. Dramatic results have been reported by parents using this supplement for ADD and hyperactivity in their children.

Some companies offering Grape Seed Extract for sale in the U.S. will sell only to health care professionals. Others allow their products to be sold over the counter. We do not know if one is more potent than another. We do know, however, that the grapes from which the Proanthocyanidin is extracted must be dark grapes with seeds.

Dimethylglycine (DMG)

It is now suspected that the same brain malfunction that leads to hyperactivity and learning disabilities may also lead to dyslogic syndrome where the ability to grasp that the concept of cause and effect is lost contributing to behavior problems (sometimes dangerous). In the 1970's, Dr. Ben Feingoid, a highly regarded pediatric allergist, reported that many hyperactive and learning disabled kids showed remarkable improvement when put on the "Feingold Natural Food, No Addi-

17

tive Diet". Feingold eliminated 3,000 additives currently found in foods and drinks. Placing a child on a natural organic foods diet will help the body rid itself of toxins and restore the right vitamins, minerals and other nutrients to the brain. This process may be enhanced with supplementation of Dimethylglycine (DMG).

Technically classified as a food, DMG is found in very small amounts in some foods, for example, rice hulls. Chemically it resembles water soluble vitamins such as the B vitamins. In an article in the *Journal of Laboratory and Clinical Medicine* (1990, 481-86) DMG is described as a "natural, simple compound with no undesirable side effects." Initially used to help autistic children, when DMG is administered, parents have reported the child's behavior improved, frustration threshold increased and speech improved within 24 hours. A Los Angeles mother started her mute autistic five year old son on DMG. The next day he was riding in the family's car when his sister began to cry. He spoke his first words, "Don't cry Kathy." His mother, stunned, nearly crashed the car. DMG is inexpensive and may improve the effectiveness of other nutrients, specifically vitamin B6 and magnesium.

Digestive Complaints

The key factors here are: food intake (timing, amount, and variety), enzyme activity, assimilation and mental state. Poor digestion indicates an overall state of imbalance.

This may be from any number of causes or it may be strictly dietary related. A simple measure to improve digestion is to take plant enzymes with every meal and stop eating late at night. Make it a rule not to eat after, say, 7:00 p.m.

Practically every disease can be traced to congestion in the bowels. If we are always snacking in between meals and then going to bed with a full stomach, the digestive system has no time to rest. Therefore, the body is required to attend to the intestinal area with a disproportionate amount of energy all of the time. This steals energy from other areas of the body also in need. A sluggish bowel inhibits brain function through lack of circulation, and reduces energy levels in general leaving a person feeling tired and irritable a lot of the time.

Taking the plant enzymes will help a great deal. The daily intake of liquid electrolyte trace minerals, fresh organic apple juice, acidophilus, flax, nutritional yeast, aged garlic extract, a green foods supplement of wheat or barley grass, and blue green algae, will help to regulate digestion and improve overall health. In addition, one may wish to consider fasting one or two days a month; this gives the body a rest. Purposeful fasting, however, is not recommended for very young children.

Garlic is noted for its restorative powers and ability to expel poisons from the body. Aged garlic extract can be taken daily.

Nutritional yeast plays a role in eliminating toxins from excess of drugs and stabilizes blood sugar rapidly. Exceptionally high in usable protein (brain food).

Lecithin nurses the brain mainly due to its broad spectrum of essential fatty acids factor (EFA).

Greens —barley, wheat grass, spirulina, chlorella, and blue green algae are excellent detoxifiers and anti oxidants.

And, of course, drinking plenty of freshly purified water is essential for total health, so drink — and have your child drink — a lot of purified water. Investigate water purification systems before buying. All systems are not created equally.

Food Therapy

Diet change has been found to be the key factor in relieving hyperactive behavior. Diet improvement results are almost immediately evident, most within one to three weeks. When behavior has normalized, maintain the improved diet to prevent reversion.

Since food sensitivities play a large part in these disorders, test common allergen foods — milk, wheat, corn, chocolate, and citrus with an elimination challenge diet; avoid all foods with sugar, dyes, colors, or additives. Eliminate all red meats (nitrates) and canned or frozen foods (too much salt). Reduce carbonated drinks.

The ongoing diet needs to be high in vegetable proteins and whole grains, with plenty of fresh fruits and vegetables, with no junk or fast foods. Include typtophan-rich foods; turkey, fish, wheat germ, yogurt, and eggs.

READ LABELS CAREFULLY. Avoid all foods with preservatives, (BHT, MSG, BHA, etc.) additives, or colors.

Other Natural Alternative Therapies

Aromatherapy

Aromatherapy utilizes the vital, aromatic essences of plant extracts, called essential oils, for healing and relaxation. It is no secret that delightful scents can make us feel better instantaneously. Molecules of odor have a direct path through the nose to the emotional part of the brain (the Limbic System). Thus emotions and thoughts are shifted immediately and create new biochemicals that bathe the bodily tissue. Smell alone can make us feel calm or irritable. There are several essential oils to consider for use with ADD. The top three would be Lavender, Peppermint and Orange.

Lavender is the most versatile and useful of all essential oils. It is instantly balancing to the central nervous system and it is also antiseptic, analgesic and anti-inflammatory. Oil of lavender is used in hospitals and nursing homes to aid sleep; its tranquilizing effects help hyperactive children rest and feel calm.

Orange is the natural tranquilizer and can have a soothing, nurturing, calming effect on hyperactive children. Mandarin or Tangerine are also sweet, soothing essential oils for infants.

Peppermint energizes with it's strong menthol content. It helps clear the mind and stabilize the emotion, and has the ability to create a feeling of calm vitality.

In choosing the appropriate oil, it is important to let the child smell the oils and make the decision as to which one is best for them. The nose-brain connection makes this choice automatically, based on the limbic system response. This process also allows the child to be in on the decision making process, thus taking on responsibility for self.

The term aromatherapy was coined in 1937 by the French chemist, Rene-Maurice Gattefosse, who, after using lavender oil to heal an accidental burn, decided to find out more about the healing properties of other essential oils, and developed aromatherapy into the science it is today. Aromatherapy is popular because of its convenience, low cost and easy accessibility.

Most essential oils are intended for topical and aromatic use only. They are not to be taken internally without the guidance of a professional. Check your local health food store, and read labels carefully; aromatic oils are not necessarily essential oils. Essential oils will be labeled as such and will generally be more expensive. Pure therapeutic grade essential oils are the best choice when the intention is to use them as the good medicine that they are.

Easy and effective ways for self care.

1. Carry the bottle of pure essential oil with you and simply inhale as often as desired. The nose-brain connection has a powerful effect on the body simply by smelling.
2. Put four drops of straight essential oil on a small piece of cotton cloth. Keep it in a pocket, in underwear, pinned to a shirt collar or place in a pillow. Recharge with 1-2 drops when needed. Lavender is excellent for this.
3. Put one drop of straight Lavender on the pillow or corner of the bed at night to aid sleeping (or have a small Lavender pillow to carry with you when you travel).
4. Make a palm bland by pouring some base oil (like jojoba or a vegetable oil), in the palm of your hand. Add one or two drops of essential oil and apply on nose, temple, neck, chest, abdomen, hands or feet. Give children a hand, feed or back massage with this blend. See which of these areas of the body is the most effective for them. One place will be their favorite. This combination of touch and oils is profound.
5. Put a diffuser in a room to cleanse the air and soothe the emotions. Fill a mini potpourri pot 3/4 with water and add 6-8 drops of essential oils.
6. Carry a mister around and mist the head and face as often as desired. Use 2 oz. of water to 4 drops of oil (such as Lavender). Shake each time you mist.
7. Baths are an ancient therapeutic healing art. This is an excellent way to balance the body, mind and emotions. After entering the bath, make the palm blend as described in #5 and apply to nose, neck, chest, abdomen. Dip a wash cloth in water and lay on your chest. Close your eyes and rest. You can add 6 or 8 drops of essential oils to the water directly. (Orange and Peppermint are too strong and should not be used as they will irritate the skin.) Lavender is best for this method.

Essential oils were among the origins of medicine and perfume. Their liquids are antiseptic and antiviral, therefore they support a healthy immune system. The fact that the liquid happens to smell, gives them the ability to soothe the mind and emotions and become a part of a package of good medicine.

Chinese Medicine

Acupuncture and Chinese herbs are ancient Chinese medical therapies documented in their effectiveness for over 2,000 years. The use of herbs in Chinese medicine is an art in and of itself. An accomplished practitioner of Chinese herbal medicine will have developed an acute insight to and awareness of the energetic qualities and healing properties of dozens of different plant, mineral, and animal medicinal substances.

A practitioner of Chinese medicine works to identify and treat patterns of imbalance and will design an individualized course of treatment based on his or her findings. A Doctor of Oriental Medicine, (D.O.), or Licensed Acupuncturist, (Lic. Ac.), usually uses both acupuncture and herbs to treat patients.

As an acupuncturist, the practitioner uses needles placed at specific points along the body's meridians, or pathways of electrical energy flow. Energy in the body is intensified in this way, letting the patient feel alive and whole again with a heightened ability to cope with stress or distraction. To have this balance restored, the patient often experiences an exhilarated sense of connectedness to his surroundings, including people. This is high energy *in focus*. Energy *out of focus*, on the other hand, can be described, in one regard, as hyperactivity, an energetic state which often makes it difficult or impossible to function effectively in one's surroundings. Hyperactivity can be regarded as lots of energy with no place to go; the energy builds until it explodes for lack of an appropriate pathway.

In Chinese medicine, energy may be seen as being deficient in some areas and excessive in others. An acupuncturist seeks to regulate this flow, using needles to send more energy to areas of deficiency (tonifying) while drawing excess out of areas in need of relief (sedation). Energy flow in the body is stimulated in this way and the optimum result is an even flowing energy rather than an erratic one. The number of sessions required to receive a balancing effect may vary according to the needs of the individual.

Peter Goldberg, Lic. Ac., a private practitioner in the state of Massachusetts says, 'The use of Acupuncture and Chinese herbs offers a gentle and natural therapeutic protocol for addressing the special needs of those with ADD. This time tested, energetic medicine supports both the physical and emotional areas of an individuals life regardless of age."

CranioSacral Therapy

CranioSacral Therapy is a gentle way of healing often yielding dramatic and profound results. Because CranioSacral Therapy directly affects the central nervous system, it is well suited for children who have attention deficit disorder or hyperactivity.

Cranio refers to the cranium, or head, and *sacral* refers to the base of the spine and tailbone. The craniosacral system is comprised of the brain and spinal cord (the central nervous system); the cerebrospinal fluid that bathes the brain and spinal cord; the surrounding membranes that enclose the brain, spinal cord and cerebrospinal fluid; and the bones of the spine and skull that house these membranes.

A practitioner of CranioSacral Therapy is able to discern the subtle rhythms of the craniosacral system by placing his or her hands on almost any part of the body and palpating the rhythm. Adjustments are made to the system through the use of a pressure equal to that of a nickel on the palm of one's hand. It is sometimes difficult to believe that this could be so, but documented research and personal testimonials leave little room for doubt or debate.

Dr. John Upledger, D.O., O.M.M., researcher and founder of The Upledger Institute in Palm Beach Gardens, Fla, insists that what is known as ADD must be considered as to its cause. Dr. Upledger, a world renown expert on CranioSacral Therapy, feels that the condition known as ADD should be considered a symptom. The cause of this symptom should be the subject for investigation. Dr. Upledger's research and previous clinical experience in the areas of ADD, hyperkinesis, and hyperactive behavior lead him to believe that there are three prominent causes that may contribute to these conditions. First, that there is dysfunction in the craniosacral system. Second, that there may be food and chemical intolerances and third, that there may be significant contribution to this condition by emotional and psychosocial causes.

In Dr. Upledgers book *Your Inner Physician and You* (one of several books by Dr. Upledger) he writes, "Our early success in the clinic [at Michigan State University] with hyperactive children was most encouraging. The hyperactive child would often fall asleep on the treatment table after we made the craniosacral system correction. Usually this problem was found at the base of the skull in the back where the head joins the neck . . . Once we released that bony 'stuckness,' the dura mater membrane system loosened and the hyperactive child began to behave more normally. Frequently dietary restrictions could then be relaxed. Food allergies significantly improved . . . If we did not find the jamming of the skull (occipital bone) forward on the neck, we observed that the hyperactivity was probably due to some other cause."

Because of the tremendous success that Dr. Upledger has had with hyperactive, autistic, and learning disabled children, the authors of this publication strongly recommend that you find out more about CranioSacral Therapy to see if it might benefit your child.

Flower Remedies

In the early 1930's the noted British physician and scientist, Dr. Edward Bach, observed that many of his patients would display emotional and psychological difficulties such as apprehension, worry, loneliness, boredom, depression, uncertainty, hopelessness or fear, prior to the onset of physical illness. He also noted these same difficulties inhibited the body's natural healing ability to prevent and/or overcome disease.

Bach devoted his life to finding out more about this. After many years of research and testing, he discovered that the homeopathic preparations of 38 flowering plants, trees, and special waters alleviated a broad range of emotional and psychological difficulties.

Homeopathic preparations of plants differ from herbal preparations of plants in the following way: Homeopathic preparations are *dilutions* of the original substance whereas herbal medicinal tinctures are *concentrations* of the original substance. To be effective, homeopathic preparations must be prepared under very strict guidelines. These guidelines are highly specific and must be adhered to without deviation. The end result is a medicine containing an infinitesimal amount of the original substance. Exactly how this works in the body has not been established. We do know, however, that deviations of infinitesimal amounts of certain substances can powerfully and adversely affect one's health — thyroid hormone for example. Unlike chemical drugs and tranquilizers, which can mask and suppress symptoms causing deeper damage as a result, the infinitesimal dosage works as a catalyst to alleviate the underlying emotional causes of stress. In this way the body is encouraged to heal itself without much further intervention.

Specific to children with learning and behavioral difficulties are certain behavioral traits and emotional characteristics. These may include, but are not limited to: making the same mistake over and over again; lack of confidence or not trying for fear of failure; daydreaming and short attention span; lack of motivation for no apparent reason; interrupted concentration due to persistent unwanted thoughts; and becoming easily discouraged.

Listed as follows are the flower remedies that have proven helpful with ADD in children:

For Repeating the Same Mistakes

CHESTNUT BUD: For children repeating the same mistake, in school, and in life. They take longer to grasp lessons.

For "Daydreamers"

CLEMATIS: For daydreamers with short attention spans. Many of their learning difficulties tend to be from the fact they are 'somewhere else' in terms of their concentration.

For the Discouraged One who "Gives Up"

GENTIAN: Used with the child that becomes discouraged and gives up too easily.

For Those Lacking Confidence

LARCH: For children who feel they are not as good or talented as others. They lack confidence and often give up in anticipation of failure.

For Persistent Unwanted Thoughts

WHITE CHESTNUT: For children that find that their concentration is hampered by persistent unwanted thoughts.

For Those Lacking Motivation

WILD ROSE: For children lacking motivation and initiative for no apparent reason.

For Stress in General

CALMING ESSENCE. A combination remedy.

Herbal Medicine

From the beginning of time plants have accompanied us as we have needed them, providing beauty, shelter, and healing they have always been there for us. Plants inspire us to begin a new life and to stick it out through the difficult times. It has been said that the wild herbs growing near us in the greatest abundance are the ones we need most for healing our lives. Therefore, if dandelions — an excellent liver tonic — are most prevalent in your location, it is possible that people living in that region are suffering from liver maladies manifesting as explosive temperament, chronic fatigue, depression, indecision, and anger. Nature always has an answer, even to the most difficult of problems; it is we who must learn to listen and see in a way that nature sees — in terms of balance.

Different herbs are indicated for different ailments, and prepared herbs, just as fresh herbs, must be combined very carefully for effectiveness and specificity. We must understand not only what we are taking, but why. Understanding this, is one of the essential first steps in treating any ailment with herbal medicines.

Certain key herbs are used in the control of hyperactivity. Valerian Root is one of the best herbs of a relaxant nature. Studies of Valerian have shown a marked increase of concentration abilities and energy levels. Hops are most commonly used for their calming effect on the nervous system and are fast acting. Skullcap is considered a natural sedative whose main purpose is to induce sleep, a necessary part of all healing. Wild Lettuce is also a sleep inducer, and lessens the excitability of the nerves and nerve centers which helps to reduce pain.

A master herbalist believes in treating people as opposed to treating diseases. They take into consideration the person's history, home life, physical and mental conditions, and their personalities. All of these will contribute to a highly individual assessment and a clear picture of what herbs are indicated for that person.

Although each case is treated separately, McDermott offers the names of 4 herbs that figure prominently when treating children with ADD. These are: Betonica, Ginkgo, Scutellaria, and Vinca minor. Emphasis is on enhancing cerebral circulation.

Cat's Claw or Una de Gato is a medicinal herb known to enhance one's immune system; act as an anti-inflammatory and improve the regulation of the digestive system. This herbal wonder has shown proof through numerous accounts of improvement in intestinal absorption. It also decreases intestinal passages of partially digestive ("leaky gut"), peptides, fungus, bacteria's and parasites, which trigger constant activation of the immune system and the resulting inflammatory response which in the case of ADD, will manifest as a brain allergy.

As one's digestive system is calmed down, his or her brain also settles down, thereby having a better chance of sorting out emotions, feelings and thoughts. This has a benefit of improving the ability to sleep and rest. As an overall benefit, a person will improve os or her productivity. In the case of a child he or she can concentrate and progress in school and have a better relationship with peers, teachers, parents, and most of all, themselves.

Other herbs that have been suggested for use with ADD and hyperactivity include: Fresh Milky Oats (Avena sativa), fresh Lemon Balm Herb (Melissa officinalis), Camomile, and dried Hawthorn fruit and flower (Crataegus bilboa). Use caution when self medicating with herbs; combining them requires a certain degree of knowledge.

If one wishes to try a singular herb for ADD - more of a self help measure - Ginkgo has been reported to restore memory to youngsters who forget things all the time, and to increase concentration and focus. Ginkgo trees live for hundreds of years and have survived for thousand of years virtually unchanged as a species. This evidence of Ginkgo's genetic integrity and longevity indicates its usefulness in brain disorders and with symptoms normally associated with aging such as impaired memory function, a common attribute of ADD. Ginkgo can be purchased at a natural food market.

ADD Co-pilots

In adolescents ADD is often accompanied by complaints of acne, digestive upset, insomnia, menstrual difficulties, melancholia, and fatigue. When considering how to treat these one should first determine whether or not these are side effects of a medication or an imbalance caused by something else. If you think the medication may be to blame, consult your physician. Never discontinue any medication without the proper authorization. Once the medication has been ruled out as the possible cause or has been discontinued under the care of a physician, you are then free to begin to explore your options for restoring balance to the body through natural means.

What follows are some of the key ingredients for a successful outcome in the end for the complaints of acne, digestive trouble, insomnia, menstrual difficulties, melancholia, and fatigue, especially as they relate to ADD in adolescents.

Acne

Keep the face and hands clean and STOP TOUCHING the face. When considering facial cleansers, choose something mild and organic, preferably plant based.

Do not wear moisturizer at night. Instead, simply cleanse the skin — gently — and then spritz with a nourishing formula of electrolyte trace minerals and herbs. Horsetail, cammomile, aloe vera, burdock root, and comfrey are good herbs for the skin. Do this for several months and begin to notice the natural glow of health shining through. A light application of carefully chosen moisturizer may be worn throughout the day. Use very little makeup and be sure to cleanse the face at night .

Understand that acne is usually related to intestinal congestion and/or hormonal imbalances along with blood impurities and excess worry and fear. To clear these underlying problems is to bring about a lasting cure.

Use grape seed extract in the capsule form and take enzyme supplements and electrolyte trace minerals on a regular basis. Steam the face with cammomile water and dot troublesome areas with tea tree oil five times daily. Eat pesticide and additive free foods, drink pure water and think happy thoughts.

An adequate supply of Omega 3's and 6's are not only helpful, but may trigger a seemingly miraculous result. Obtain these nutrients from flax seed meal, borage oil, and oil of evening primrose. Use essential oil of lavender in the following way: sprinkle a couple of drops onto your hands and rub the hands together. Then press the hands onto the face (avoiding the eye area). The molecules of essential oil rapidly penetrate the skin and go to work to heal it.

Insomnia, Menstrual Difficulties, and Melancholia

These imbalances reflect a tendency towards excess in two possible directions: expansive or contractive. Mental state is an issue here. That is to say, self-image plays a part. Also, nutrient intake or lack thereof plays another. A lack of nutrients can create an artificially induced miserable mental state. A worried mind might keep a person awake all night. Essential oil of lavender will help, but for a lasting effect balance must be restored through the use of liquid minerals and other supplements. Minerals are absolutely essential when melancholia or depression is present. The minerals must be taken regularly for 4-6 months before any lasting results can be expected because during the first 4-6 months the electrolyte minerals work to cleanse the system. Heavy metal deposits are cleared out at this time as well. This is hard work for the body, and many times a "healing crisis" will occur where negative emotions stored in the cells will be released. When this happens, certain illnesses could appear as toxins work their way out of the body. Recent research has suggested that calcium and magnesium citrate are useful in detoxifying the body from aluminum poisoning.

Acupuncture treatments and CranioSacral Therapy sessions will help restore balance. Accupressure points can quickly and effectively relieve menstrual cramps. Ask someone who knows about these points to teach you how to use them. Valerian may be taken before bedtime to aid sleep, and oil of bergamot diffused in a room helps to lift depression. Learn, learn and learn, and be thirsty for knowledge.

Fatigue

Fatigue may indicate many things, but most of all fatigue points to a congested liver, also to digestive trouble and perhaps kidney weakness as well. Fatigue is often accompanied by anger and sadness, emotions related to the liver and the kidneys, respectively.

Most of the same principles apply: Take liquid electrolyte minerals and green foods supplements such as barley and wheat grass. Maintain an adequate supply of essential fatty acids including Omega 3's and 6's. Help strengthen your child's digestive system by feeding higher quality food and not too late at night. Encourage your child to rest, stretch and breathe deeply. Laugh with your child. Play with your child.

Use foot reflexology to help bring new life to overworked organs. Foot reflexology is easy to use, costs nothing and really works! Kidney points are located on the bottom of the feet, just below and to the middle of the pad beneath the big toe. Press deeply and rub. A sharp pain will be felt if there is congestion. Rub every day until there is no more sharp pain. Then the kidney problem will be reduced. Do the same for the liver. The liver point is located on the outside edge of the right foot from the bottom of the pinky toe down to about the middle of the foot. Refer to Mildred Carter's book, *Helping Yourself With Foot Reflexology*. This is a great way to help yourself and your children at home.

Fatigue can also be related to chemical sensitivities from cleaning products, pesticides, and food additives or candida albicans. The same goes for irritability, allergies, chronic sinusitis and a whole host of other ailments. Doris Rapp, M.D, author of *Is This Your Child?* and William Crook, M.D. author of *The Yeast Connection* and *Help for the Hyperactive Child* are two authorities on the subject of food allergies, candida, and chemical sensitivities. Their work is so relevant, thorough and impressive that we wish simply to refer you to them and let you investigate further for yourself.

The Integrated Approach

A lot of information has been given to you in these pages. Sometimes it is difficult to know where to begin. We suggest that you begin with the thing that grabs your attention — what stands out to you, what seems to make the most sense. Next step is to design an approach that works for your family.

We suggest starting with the things that may offer immediate gratification such as CranioSacral Therapy and Grape Seed Extract or Pycnogenol. Then add to this the liquid electrolyte trace minerals and stick with those for at least 6 months before making any judgments. Add zinc, enzymes, green foods, aged garlic extract and essential fatty acids. Use the flower remedies as needed and enjoy the pleasures and benefits of aroma therapy (but not in conjunction with the flower remedies as strong odors may cancel out the homeopathic medicine.) Use foot reflexology herbal medicine and acupuncture. Breathe deeply. Play, laugh and sing with your child. Another benefit to many children with ADD is martial arts. We like Aikido because it is a way of peace, teaching people to live in harmony with themselves and in the world with others. But most important of all — enjoy life! There are no substitutions for joy and love. Go on, be free, and wake up singing.

Bibliography

Balch, James F., M.D., and Phyllis A. Balch, C.N.C. *Prescription for Nutritional Healing.* Garden City Park, Avery Publishing Group Inc., 1993

Beinfield, Harriet, L. Ac., and Efrem Korngold, L. Ac., O.M.D. *Between Heaven and Earth, A Guide to Chinese Medicine,* New York, Ballantine Books, 1991

Carlson, Richard, Ph.D., and Benjamin Shield, editors. *Healers on Healing,* Los Angeles, Jeremy P. Tarcher, Inc., 1989

Caner, Mildred. *Helping Yourself With Foot Reflexology,* West Nyack, NY, Parker Publishing Company, 1969

Fischer-Rizzi, Susanne. *Complete Aromatherapy Handbook, Essential Oils for Padiant Health,* New York, Sterling Publishing, 1990.

Fukuoka, Masanobu. *The Natural Way of Farming,* Tokyo and New York, Japan Publications, Inc., 1985.

Garber, Marian & Stephen, *Beyond Ritalin,* Random House, 1996

Hay, Louise. *You Can Heal Your Life,* Carson, CA, Hay House, Inc., 1984

Martlew, Gillian, N.D. *Electrolytes, The Spark of Life,* Nature's Publishing, Ltd., 1994

Mendelsohn, Robert, M.D. *How to Raise a Healthy Child in Spite of Your Doctor,* New York, Ballantine, 1984

Page, Linda Rector, *Healthy Healing,* 1995

Rapp, Doris, M.D. *Is This Your Child?* New York, William Morrow and Company, Inc., 1991

Tierra, Michael, C.A., N.D. *The Way of Herbs,* New York, Simon and Schuster, Inc., 1990

Upledger, John E., D.O., O.M.M. *Your Inner Pysician and You,* Berkeley, CA, North Atlantic Books, 1991.

Resource Directory

ADHD NUTRITIONAL KIT. Developed by child psychiatrists, used worldwide, this select group of nutritional products combined effect, has been found to be a helpful adjunct to educational and medical programs. Makes possible reducing or discontinuing Ritalin or Cylert. It includes, Pure Deanol, Ginkgo Bilboa, O2B1 (Thiamin Boost), B/12/Folic Acid Boost, ALUMIN/OUT. Products are sublingual & easy to take. (30% discount by mentioning this book) EN GARDE HEALTH PRODUCTS, 7702 Bldg. #10, Balboa Blvd., Van Nuys, CA 91406 (800)-955-4MED (818-901-8505) Fax (818-786-4699) Send #10 SASE for 44 pg. catalog.

IMMUNE SYSTEM SUPPORT. This company provides a nutrient rich powdered "green" drink high in amino acids, vitamins and anti-oxidants; aged garlic extract to fight heavy metal poisoning, bacteria and infectious disease; "friendly" strains of intestinal bacteria, necessary for colon health; and Ginkgo Biloba for mental health. Kyolic, Kyo-Green, Kyo-Dophilus WAKUNAGA OF AMERICA, 23501 Madero, Mission Viejo, CA 92691 (800)-825-7888.

DIGESTIVE ENZYMES. This all natural formula contains all the necessary enzymes for digestion throughout the intestinal tract. These capsules are highly bioavailable and absorbable. Contains protease, amylase, lipase and cellulase in powder form. Taking enzymes whenever cooked or processed foods are eaten will guard against food allergies and their associated emotional effects. PROZYME PRODUCTS, LTD. 6600 N. Lincoln Ave., Suite 312, Lincolnwood IL 60645 (800)-522-5537 call Debra Casey for information.

ESSENTIAL FATTY ACID (EFA) BALANCER. As necessary ingredients for proper cellular neurotransmitter function in the brain and throughout the body, Omega-3 EFAs must be balanced with Omega-6 EFAs. Flax is the richest source of Omega-3 with a good balance of Omega-6. Fortified Flax and Power Pack Energy Drink Mix can be sprinkled on cereal and sandwiches or mixed with juice or water.. OMEGA-LIFE, INC. PO Box 208, Brookfield, WI 53008-0208 (800)-EAT-FLAX (328-3529).

LIQUID CRYSTALLOID ELECTROLYTE MINERALS. Trace-Lyte is a crystalloid (smallest form) electrolyte formula that helps keep cells strong, balance pH, facilitate removal of toxins and provide the body's life force. If extra magnesium is required, Cal-Lyte offers a 1:1 ratio of calcium/magnesium with boron to assist absorption. Also available is Total-Lyte which increases mental efficiency, improves concentration, nourishes the brain and combats school fatigue.. NATURE'S PATH, INC., PO Box 7862, Venice, FL 34287-7862 (800)-326-5772.

MIGHTY GREENS. This new product is a very strong combination of amino acids, anti-oxidants and other nutrients that support the immune system and all the body functions. Mighty Greens is a blend of wheat, barley, rye and oat grass along with spirulina and chlorella. Also included in the formula are 22 other support herbs including ginkgo biloba, ginseng, and grape skin extract. PINES INTERNATIONAL, PO Box 1107, Lawrence KS 66044 (800)-697-4637.

FLOWER ESSENCES, HERBS, AND HERBAL MASSAGE THERAPIES. These treatment modalities treat various types of emotional imbalances, and personality/mental difficulties gently, safely and effectively. Healing Herbs™ is composed of 38 English essences based on the writings of a noted British physician over 60 years ago. FES Quintessentials™ is composed of 103 North American flower essences. Herbal flower oils and Self Help Creme™ are available for massage and skin care. Available through BAYSIDE QUALITY PRODUCTS LTD. (888) 724-5489.

BRAIN FUNCTION SUPPORT. The link between nutrition and brain function has been confirmed by numerous studies which show that deficiencies in certain essential fatty acids may be tied to specific behavioural traits consistent with ADHD and other learning difficulties. Efalex™ Focus provides High DHA Tuna Oil, GLA rich Efamol Evening Primrose Oil, and powerful antioxidants Thyme Oil and Vitamin E. Call toll-free 1-888-EFALEX-1. EFAMOL NUTRACEUTICALS, INC., 23 Dry Dock Avenue, Boston, MA 02210. Email www.efamol.com.

TRANSFORMATION FORMULAS. CalmZyme herbal formula helps in controlling the effects of various nervous system disorders including hyperactivity. Protein that is not broken down by the digestive system, cannot be absorbed. Protein deficiency is a contributor to ADD. PureZyme protease enzymes break down protein and increase its absorption. DigestZyme is an enzyme complex that enhances digestion. TRANSFORMATION, 2900 Wilcrest, Suite 220, Houston, TX 77042 (800) 777-1474.

MINERALS & HERBS FOR YOUR FACE. Providing crystalloid, electrolyte trace minerals and herbs including Aloe, Horsetail (silica), Chamomile, Comfrey and Burdock Root. Skin Lyte™ is an excellent treatment for acne, rashes, dermatitis, eczema and other skin ailments. NATURE'S PATH, INC., PO Box 7862, Venice, FL 34287-7862 (800)-326-5772.

FOCUS FORMULA. Includes fresh Oats Seed, Skullcap, Hawthorn fruit & flower, Ginkgo leaf, Lemon Balm. Alcohol-free Focus Formula Glycerite contains fresh Oats, Skullcap, Lemon Balm in vegetable glycerine and distilled water with solid extraction of Hawthorn fruit. HERBALIST & ALCHEMIST, INC. PO BOX 553, Broadway, NJ 08808 (800)-611-8235.

UPLEDGER INSTITUTE. (CRANIOSACRAL THERAPY) Learn more about CranioSacral Therapy and how it can help ease the symptoms of A.D.D. naturally, without medications. Intensive programs for children with A.D.D. and learning disabilities are available. Call for information and/or to order an international directory of practitioners. THE UPLEDGER INSTITUTE HEALTHPLEX CLINICAL SERVICES, 11211 Prosperity Farms Rd., D-223, Palm Beach Gardens, FL 33410-3487 (407) 622-4706.

HOMEOPATHIC REMEDIES. Healing begins with cleansing. The Newton #1 DETOXIFIER formula stimulates excretion of toxins by the liver and kidneys, spleen & colon. Taken in combination with the Newton #29 BOWEL DISCOMFORT, normal digestive and intestinal processes are enhanced (crucial for restoration of children's health). For hyperactivity SIMILIG #71 HYPERACTIVITY formula is available over-the-counter. NEWTON, 2360 Rockaway Ind. Blvd., Conyers, GA 30207 (800)-448-7256 FAX (800)-760-5550 Email: newtrmdy@avana.net.

MEGAFOOD ZINC. Mother Nature is used for growing minerals to create highly potent MegaFood Whole Food Concentrates. A unique process converts isolated USP minerals into a nutrient dense complex similar to natural whole food, making them among the most bioavailable of all supplements on the market. Your body will feel the difference with MegaFood Zinc. BIO SAN LABORATORIES, INC. PO Box 325, Derry, NH 03038 (800)-258-5014.

PROTEIN FOODS AND SUGAR SUBSTITUES. Systemic yeast infections from antibiotics destroys the inner ecosystem of the digestive tract creating nutritional deficiences. These products can help. *Kefir* is a high protein, nutrient rich food that contains minerals, B vitamins, natural tryptophan (that promotes a calming effect). *Stevia* is a natural herbal dietary supplement that replaces sugar and aspartame. *EcoRenew* sugar-free wafer treat containing friendly bacteria. BODY ECOLOGY, 1266 W. Paces Ferry Rd., Suite 505, Atlanta GA 30327 (800)-478-3842.

EFA AND GLA SOURCES. Omega-3 essential fatty acids (EFAs) are required for brain and nervous system development. Flax and fish oil are rich sources of omega-3 EFAs. Omega-6 fatty acids are also important for health. Borage oil and Evening Primrose Oil contain nutritionally important omega-6 EFA and Gamma-Linolenic Acid (GLA). The Total EFA is a nutritionally complete and balanced combination of omega-3 and omega-6 EFAs from certified organic flax oil, borage oil and fish oil. HEALTH FROM THE SUN, PO Box 840, Sunapee, NH 03782 (800)-447-2249.

AANGAMIK DMG. DMG is a naturally occurring amino acid, a product of cellular metabolism. FoodScience has 5 U.S. patents on DMG and AANGAMIK DMG which is a foil-wrapped chewable tablet recommended by Dr. Bernard Rimland, foremost authority on Autism. Many parents have used DMG successfully in treating ADD and ADHD conditions in their children. FOODSCIENCE LABORATORIES, 20 New England Dr., Essex Junction, VT 05453 (800)-874-9444.

ALL NATURAL BROAD-SPECTRUM MICRONUTRIENTS. The stresses of increasing micronutrient deficiencies in our diet can impair the immune system resulting in many kinds of dysfunction. Ocean plants (seaweed & kelp) naturally concentrate nature's richest source of chelated minor trace minerals, including iodine, vitamins, and other complex micronutrients. MICRO-MAX in capsule form, is a potent nutritional aid that will help the bioavailability of your entire dietary program. SOURCE, INC. 101 Fowler Rd., N. Branford, CT 06471 (800)-232-2365 or (203)-488-6400.

AMINO ACID SUPPLEMENT FOR KIDS. For many, hyperactive behavior and learning disorders can be addressed by supplying the cells with the proper nutrient mix. *Kids Plex Jr.* is a complete, balanced nutritional supplement high in amino acids recognized by experts as "the primary building blocks of human life." *Kids Plex Jr.* has 100% of the RDA of vitamins and nutrients needed by a growing child. The powdered form is easy to mix in juice or sprinkled on food. NATURADE, P.O. Box 474, Dallas, TX 75370 (800)-933-7539.

DIETARY SUPPLEMENT BAR. Attention™ is a delicious dietary supplement bar designed to enhance attention span and concentration. Essential fatty acids, phospholipids, specific vitamins, minerals and botanical compounds, are provided in a unique gluco-regulatory (blood glucose) delivery system without artificial sweeteners. METABOLIC RESPONSE MODIFIERS, 2633 West Coast Highway, Suite B, Newport Beach, CA 92663 (800)-948-6296; Website: www.metamode.com

LAVENDER PILLOW & MEDICINE TIN ESSENTIAL OILS. Lavender is the #1 balancing oil to the central nervous system. The Oil Lady Aromatherapy supplies The Lavender Pillow which is 100% cotton, 8'x10' and comes with instructions and a 4 ml. bottle of pure lavender. The Medicine Tin is a self care kit for the home for making palm blends. It includes Lavender, Tea Tree, Peppermint, Eucalyptus, Orange pure essential oils, Jojoba base oil, Lavender Mist, Organic cotton cloth and guide book. Audio tapes also available. Oil Lady Aromatherapy, P.O. Box 10205, Naples, FL 34101-0205 (941) 263-3451 Fax (941) 263-0898.

CELLULAR DETOXIFICATION AND SUPPORT. Homeovitics for clearing, cellular detoxification and support. A 48 day program is available as a Protocol Pak to initiate a natural approach to ADD. The Protocol Pak is used to cleanse the body of cellular toxins, such as chemicals and metals which are a predisposing factor to ADD. Homeovitic formulations are available from your health care professional. For information: HVS LABORATORIES, 3427 Exchange Ave., Naples, FL 34104 (800) 521-7722 Web: http://www.hvslabs.com.

TASTY OMEGA-3 PRODUCT. *Essential Balance, Jr.*, for children with A.D.H.D., is a tasty blend of essential fatty acids which contains a scientifically formulated blend of flax, sunflower, pumpkin, borage and sesame oils. Omega is the only company that has organic coconut oil, DHA from algae or marine source and organic sesame oil both used in ADHD and autism diet therapy. OMEGA NUTRITION, 6515 Aldrich Rd., Bellingham, WA 98226 (800) 661-3529

DAKOTA FLAX GOLD. All natural edible flax seed, high in lignans, use over cereal, on salads, in soups, or in juice. Low in cadmium, better tasting. Available with grinder (seeds must be ground for full nutritional value). Flax is also available in capsule form. S.A.S.E. for sample. HEINTZMAN FARMS, RR2 Box 265, Onaka, SD 57466 (800) 333-5813. HTTP://www.worldprofit.com/health/mbflax.htm.

Recommended Reading

Allergies and the Hyperactive Child, Doris Rapp, MD, Pediatrician

Is This Your Child? Doris Rapp, MD, Pediatrician

Body, Mind and Sugar, E.M. Abrahamson, MD & A.W. Pezet

Healthy Choices Conquers Disease, Jo-Anne Rohn

Solving the Puzzle of Your Hard -To-Raise Child, Dr.Wm. G. Crook

Help for the Hyperactive Child, Dr. Wm. G. Crook

Healthier Children, Barbara Kahan

Low Blood Sugar, Carlton Fredericks, Ph.D.

Sweet & Dangerous, John Yudkin, M.D.

Beyond Ritalin, Marian & Stephen Garber

Is This Your Child's World?, Doris J. Rapp, M.D., Pediatrition

Why Can't My Child Behave?, Jane Hersey

Developmental Delay Registry (Newsletter), 1-301-652-2263

OTHER BOOKS AVAILABLE FROM SAFE GOODS

★*OVER 50 LOOKING 30! The Secrets of Staying Young.* $ 9.95
How to become wrinkle resistant and fight the signs of aging.
★*All Natural Anti-Aging Skin Care* $ 4.95
The newest information on keeping your skin young.
★*The All Natural Anti-Aging Diet* $ 4.95
Eat lots, Stay slim and avoid old age diseases
★*The A.D.D. and A.D.H.D. DIET!* $ 9.95
look at contributing factors and natural treatments for ADD/ADHD.
★*Put Hemorrhoids and Constipation Behind You* $14.95
A natural healing guide for easy, quick and lasting relief.
★*The Humorous Herbalist* $14.95
Practical guide to leaves, flowers, roots, bark and other neat stuff
★*Super Nutrition for Animals (Birds Too!)* $12.95
Healthy advice for Dogs, Cats, Ferrets, Horses and Birds.
★*A Guide To A Naturally Healthy Bird* $ 8.95
Nutritional information for parrots and other caged birds.
★*Plain English Guide to your PC* $ 8.95
The computer book that tells it better and tells it in English.
★*The Brain Train* $ 4.95
How to keep our brain healthy and wise (for children).
★*Natural Solutions to Sexual Dysfunction* $ 9.95
Natural alternatives to drug therapy for sexual problems.
★*Growth Hormone, The Methuselah Factor* $12.95
Reverse human aging naturally.
★*The Backseat Flyer* $ 9.95
Plane Sense about flying as a passenger

Order Line (800)-903-3837
Safe Goods Publishing
PO Box 36, E. Canaan CT 06024
860-824-5301
www.animaltails.com